Fast and Affordable Makeup:

Six Steps for Getting Pretty in a Pinch

E. W. PERTI

To my friends, who always made me feel like a
professional makeup artist, long before I was one!

CONTENTS

Introduction

As an artist and writer, I have many options for creative outlet, but makeup has always been my favorite medium because it has such range. We can wear makeup to make ourselves look better and therefore, feel better... or to make ourselves feel better and therefore, look better! We can also wear makeup to express ourselves or stand out in a crowd. Or, we can wear makeup to fit in or play a role! But before we can get into all the different things that can be done with makeup, we have to learn the basics.

That's where this book comes in! I'm so happy you chose to start here — or make a stop here — on your makeup journey. Out of all the ways you can learn about makeup, starting with this book will help you learn the fundamentals in a clear and succinct way! Of course, the internet — especially social media — has endless information about makeup... but it has so much, in fact, that it's hard to know where to start! But don't worry — I know where to start!

Additionally, much of the information online is shared by influencers who are paid to endorse certain products that are often not as great as they're touted to be. Also, many beauty influencers are great at doing makeup on themselves, but might not have much experience doing makeup on other people! As a special event makeup artist, I have over ten years' worth of experience applying makeup on over a thousand *different* faces! For this book, I've boiled down all my knowledge into nice, neat, easy-to-absorb little chapters.

Although my experience is with special event makeup, my passion is natural-looking makeup that helps women feel like the prettiest version of themselves instead of someone unrecognizable. In this book, I am including the most important, highest-impact steps for making yourself look polished and pretty while still looking like yourself! I am *not* including time-consuming steps or products that are unnecessary for an everyday makeup look. Keeping things simple will not only save you time, but also money because you won't be purchasing unnecessary products. In fact, you may find that you already have several of the supplies you need to get started!

Before we get to the fun stuff, I have one more thing to say. Although I consider myself to be an experienced makeup artist, I always try to keep in mind that makeup is an *art*. There is a lot of science involved in makeup, but it is not *hard science*. And, to that end, there is usually more than one effective approach to any makeup goal. Additionally, people have a wide range of aesthetic preferences (.i.e., what is considered beautiful). So, it's quite possible that something you read in this book might go against something you've heard somewhere else. That doesn't mean either of us are wrong — it's just a reminder than makeup is a highly-individualized art form! You can try it my way, her way, his way, etc... but ultimately you will find what works for you!

In the next chapter you will find the supplies that you will need to complete the 6-Step process that I outline in this book. Do yourself a favor and don't buy anything new until after you've read all the chapters!

CHAPTER ONE

What You Will Need

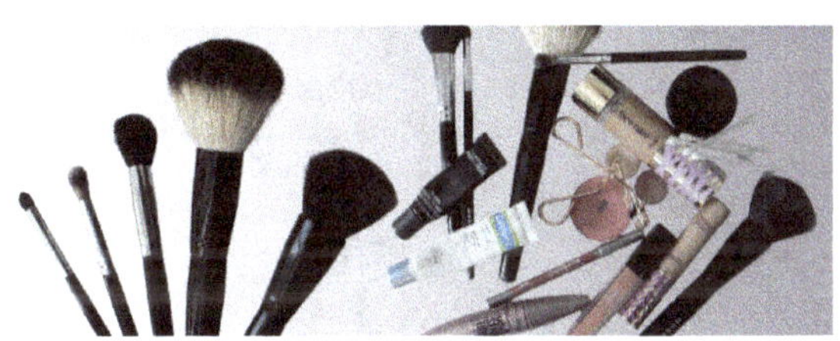

<u>**For each item, find more details in the corresponding chapter.**</u>

Step 1: Lashes
- ✓ An eyelash curler (unless your lashes are already naturally curled)
- ✓ Mascara
- ✓ Cotton swab sticks (such as Q-Tips)
- ✓ A gentle eye cream

Step 2: Eye Shadow

- ✓ Nude shadows with either warm, cool, or neutral undertones
- ✓ Small and medium eyeshadow brushes

Step 3: Foundation
- ✓ The foundation of your choice
- ✓ A large, densely-bristled brush

Step 4: Concealer
- ✓ Under-eye concealer
- ✓ Blemish concealer

Step 5: Blush
- ✓ Blush (or blush palette) of your choice
- ✓ Blush brush (if using powder blush)

(Step 5.5: Setting Powder — optional)
- ✓ Setting powder of your choice

Step 6: Lip Color
- ✓ Lip liner (*optional*)
- ✓ Lip color of your choice

Optional finishing touches:
- ✓ Brow gel
- ✓ Setting spray
- ✓ Blotting papers

CHAPTER TWO

Skincare

Taking care of your skin and wearing makeup go hand in hand. If you don't already have a makeup routine, I suggest you take a few days to focus on starting one before you tackle these new makeup steps. Although it can take time to see the benefits of a skin care routine and the results are not always as dramatic as what can be achieved with makeup, it is still very important. Caring for your skin has compounding benefits, especially when it comes to makeup. If you have clearer, smoother skin, you won't feel as though you need as much makeup. Additionally, makeup looks better on smoother skin than it does on dry, rough, textured, sun-damaged skin.

Although expensive laser treatments and prescription skincare systems can give you great results *if you need them,* your routine does not need to be expensive or complicated. Because this is not a book on skincare, I'm not going to get very in-depth. But, in order for your makeup to sit nicely on your skin, you should at least do the following simple steps daily.

THE BARE MINIMUM OF SKIN CARE

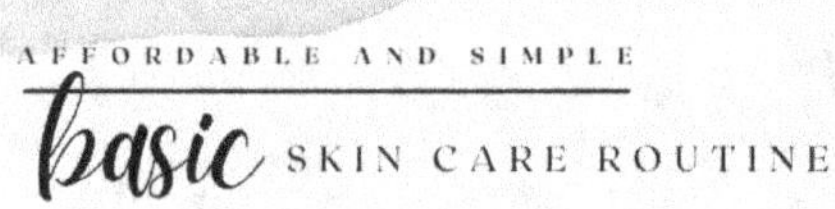

AFFORDABLE AND SIMPLE

basic SKIN CARE ROUTINE

This is all you need from teens to mid-twenties!
After that, these are the basics, and you can add other
products under the direction of a skincare professional.

morning	*evening*
1. Wash with a mild cleanser, such as *Cetaphil Gentle Skin Cleanser* 2. Apply an oil-free moisturizer with broad spectrum SPF 30 or higher such as, *CeraVe AM Facial Moisturizing Lotion with Sunscreen*	1. Remove eye makeup with a gentle makeup remover such as *Neutrogena Oil-Free Eye Makeup Remover* 2. Follow up with the same cleanser you used in the morning 3. Apply a nighttime moisturizer such as *CeraVe PM Facial Moisturizing Lotion*

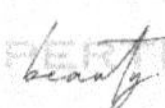

DON'T PICK IT!

Do not pick at the surface of your skin! Try your best to allow blemishes to go through their natural cycle and heal on their own. Picking at them damages your skin and makes it much more likely to scar. Not to mention… an oozing pimple is impossible to cover with concealer! If you really must pop a pimple, wait until it has come to a head, and do it at night before bed so it has time to calm down before you need to go anywhere or apply makeup.

CHAPTER THREE

Choosing Colors

When it comes to choosing makeup shades that flatter your skin, understanding your *undertone* is important. Makeup colors fall into three color categories — warm, cool, and neutral. These categories come into play when choosing your foundation, blush, and cheek colors.

* * *

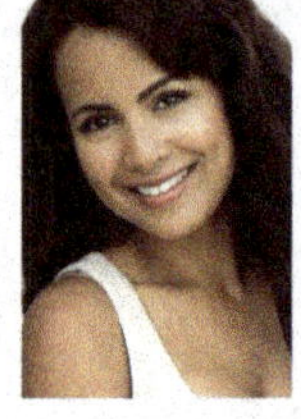
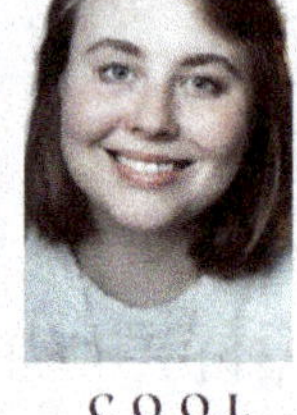
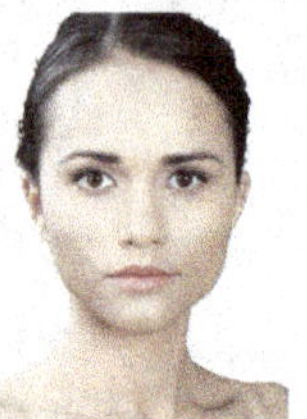
FIND YOUR
undertone
WARM
COOL
NEUTRAL

WARM UNDERTONES

Warm undertones have a golden, yellow, or peachy base. People with warm undertones often have skin that tans easily in the sun, and gold jewelry looks amazing on them.

For **cheek color**, people with warm skin tones look fabulous in shades with peachy undertones, such as *Milani's Luminoso* or terracotta undertones, like *Milani's Rose D'Oro*. These will create a sun-kissed glow that complementing their natural warmth.

For **eyeshadow**, people with warm undertones can use neutral as well as warm tones for a more natural look. *NYX Professional Makeup Ultimate Color Shadow Palette in Warm Neutrals* is a perfect option.

For **lip colors**, look for words like *warm, peach, and coral* in the description of the color. *E.L.F. O FACE Satin Lipstick in Standing Ovation* or *Cover Girl Clean Lip Color Lipstick* in *Darling Kiss, Maple Glaze* or *Warm Taupe* are a beautiful options for people with warm skin tones.

* * *

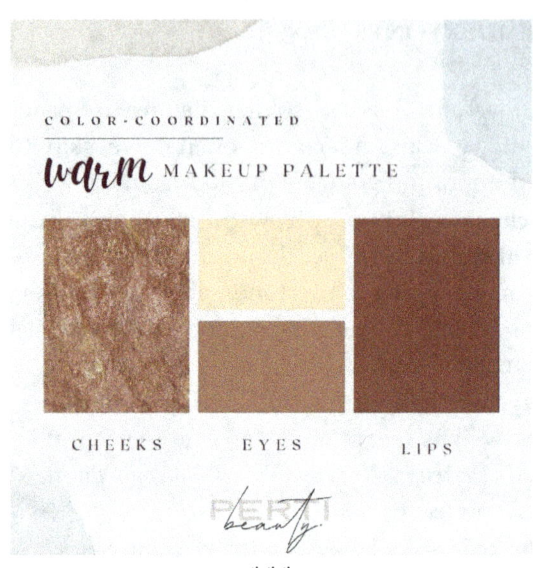
COLOR·COORDINATED
warm MAKEUP PALETTE
CHEEKS   EYES   LIPS
PERTI
beauty.

***

COOL UNDERTONES

Cool undertones have pink, red, or blueish shades, and are often fair-skinned.

For **cheek color**, choose shades with true pink or rosy undertones, such as *Milani's Baked Blush in Dolce Pink* or *Petal Primavera*.

For **lip color**, people with cool undertones look great in rose and berry colors, such as *e.l.f. O FACE Satin Lipstick in Effortless or Shameless*.

Eyeshadows in grayish browns look natural and flattering. *Morphe's 18CT Matte Essentials Artistry Palette* is a perfect option with plenty of nude cool colors to choose from.

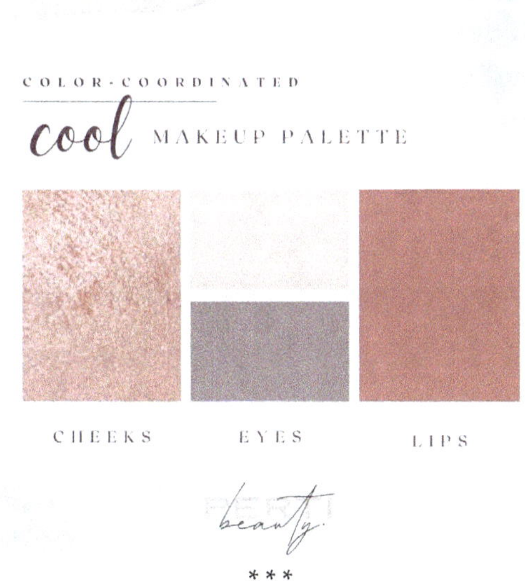

* * *

NEUTRAL UNDERTONES

If neither the warm nor the cool category sound quite like you, then you probably have neutral undertones! Neutral undertones strike a balance between yellow and blue. People with neutral undertones can often wear a wide range of colors! Neutrals can pull off both warm and cool shades without looking washed out. Multicolor palettes for each type of makeup are a great investment if you want to have fun and keep your options open. Here are some of my favorites:

Blush — *Morphe's Complexion Pro Face Palettes* in for fair (*8F*), medium (*8M*), tan (*8T*), rich (*8R*), and deep (*8D*) skin tones.

Eyeshadow — *Colour Pop's 11:11 Pressed Powder Palette* or *Morphe's 18T Truth or Bare Artistry Palette*

Lipcolor — *Jerome Alexander New Again Lipstick Palette* (in *Nude, Sexy Lips,* or *Sumptuous Shades*)

* * *

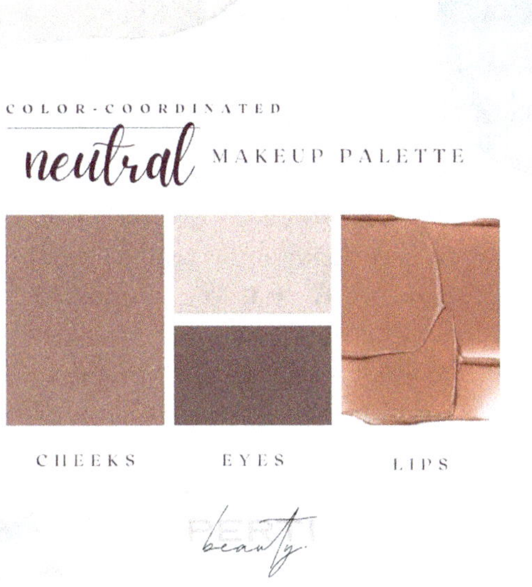
COLOR-COORDINATED
neutral MAKEUP PALETTE
CHEEKS   EYES   LIPS
beauty

* * *

COORDINATING COLORS

Knowing your undertone helps you create harmony in your look. If your undertone falls neatly into either the *warm* or *cool* categories, your best bet is to stick to colors from your category.

If you have a *neutral* skin undertone, you can wear colors from any category, but try not to mix undertone categories in the same look! Choosing colors with the same undertone for your eyes, cheeks, and lips will create a harmonious, polished look. For example, if you plan on wearing a warm red lip color, then I recommend sticking with colors from the warm family on your cheeks and eyes, too.

Also, as a general rule of thumb, if you want to go with a bold or dark color, only do it one area. For example, if you're doing dark eyeshadow, keep your cheek and lip colors pretty tame. Doing bold colors in more than one area tends to look like stage makeup.

* * *

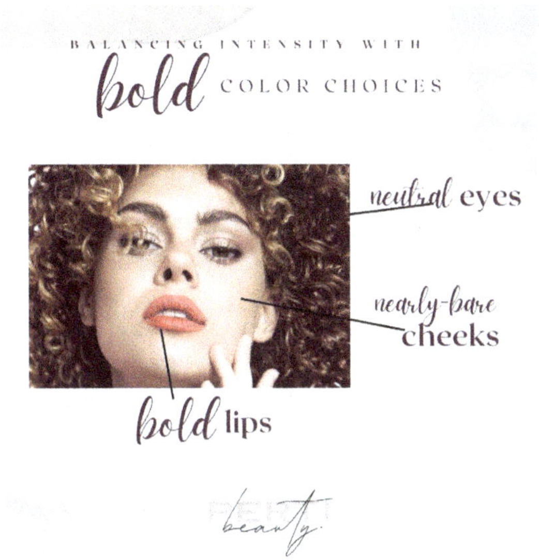

BALANCING INTENSITY WITH
bold COLOR CHOICES

CHAPTER FOUR

Step 1: Lashes

If I only have time to do one makeup step, I do my lashes! In my opinion, accentuating lashes provides the biggest payoff.

LASHES FIRST?!

Yes, lashes first! I know it is probably not where you were expecting to start. But, despite what you see on social media, makeup artists often start with eyes first! Doing your mascara and eyeshadow before you do any skin makeup allows you to easily clean up any messes you make during the eye makeup process without ruining the work you've already done on your skin. Still not sure what I mean? You might just have to trust me on this one! It will make sense by the end of this chapter.

* * *

CURLING LASHES

If you're going to curl your lashes (which I recommend for most people) you need to do it before applying mascara and eyeshadow. I first learned the power of curling my stick-straight lashes in 12th grade. One day, I decided to play with my mom's eyelash curler. I'd seen her use it in her routine countless times, but… why would I do the same thing as my mom?! Even though she did wear a little makeup every day, she wasn't in the habit of doling out beauty advice, because she always focused on nurturing my creativity and kindness. (Thanks, mom!)

Anyway, that 1980's Revlon contraption was magical. Suddenly, I had people complimenting my "pretty eyes" for the first time in my life, even though I'd been wearing mascara since 8th grade.

Straight lashes have a certain, sultry kind of beauty, but if you want to make your eyes really stand out and look bigger, curling your lashes is the way to go. Even if your lashes naturally curve up, you would probably benefit from curling them even more at the base for an extra lift.

Why does this have such an effect when you still have the same number of lashes whether their straight or curled? Well, when lashes are straight, people looking directly at you don't have a great angle to see how long or thick they may be. Curling lashes up so that they fan out in contrast to your eyelid really shows them off… especially when you add mascara!

Just make sure you always curl your lashes before applying mascara. Curling lashes with mascara already on will likely make the lashes look chunky and clumpy… and could rip several lashes out!

Check out the difference between uncurled lashes and curled lashes.

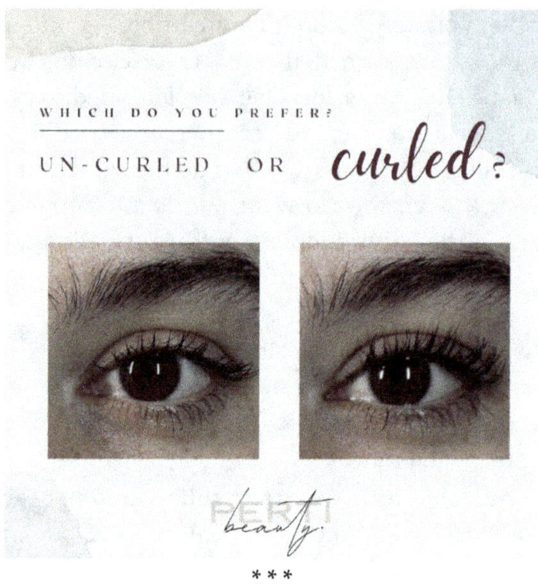

***

HOW TO CURL YOUR LASHES

There are many options for lash curlers, but I love *e.l.f.'s Pro Eyelash Curler* for it's low price and spring-loaded handle.

For the most lift and curl, try to get the curler as close to the root of your lashes as possible. Squeeze slowly at first to make sure you don't feel a pinch. If you don't feel a pinch, squeeze down hard on the curler. You do not need to squeeze for long time. It's more about the pressure than the time you hold it.

Essentially, you want to make a series of crimps in your lashes that work together to create the curl. After clamping at the base of your lashes, release the curler, slide up the lashes a tiny bit and clamp down again. Continue this process in tiny increments until you reach the tip. The number of times you need to clamp down will depend on how well your lashes accept the crimp and how long they are. If you have short lashes, you may only be able to clamp the curler once or twice, but aim for at least twice so your lashes don't just make a 90-degree angle.

* * *

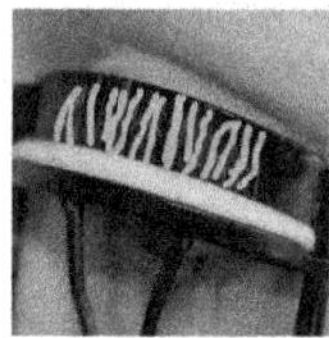
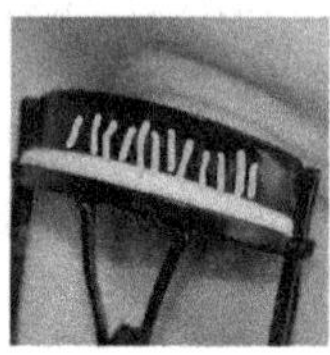
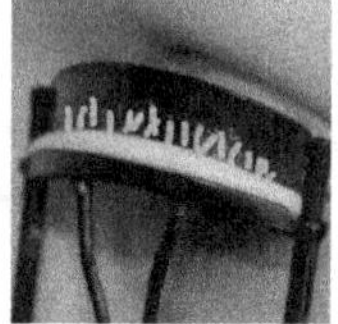

HOW TO *curl* YOUR LASHES

1. CLAMP AS CLOSE TO THE LASH BASE AS POSSIBLE

2. CLAMP IN THE MIDDLE OF THE LASHES

3. CLAMP JUST UNDER THE TIPS OF THE LASHES

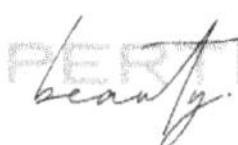

Pro tip: To help curl lashes faster (i.e. not have to clamp as many times) blast your metal curler with a hair dryer for 5-10 seconds. Just make sure to test the temperature on the inside of your wrist before you apply it to your eyes so you don't burn yourself!

MASCARA

Mascara comes in different formulas and with a variety of brushes to meet your specific needs. The first main category is based on your goal for your lashes: **lengthening, volumizing, curling,** or any combination of the three. Note: "Curling" mascaras create more of a lift than a curl, but can be a great option if your lashes already have some curl. Once you decide what your goal is, you can further narrow your selection by durability: **washable** (i.e. water-soluble) or

waterproof.

WASHABLE MASCARA

If you have naturally curled lashes and don't expect to cry, sweat, or get caught in a downpour, **washable** will work for you. Washable mascara comes off easily at the end of the day with eye makeup remover or even a gentle face wash. You may need to stick with washable if you have a very sensitive eye area.

WATERPROOF MASCARA

If you have naturally straight or only slightly-curved lashes, **waterproof** mascara does the best job of maintaining your work with the lash curler. Think of it as hairspray for your lashes (without the stinging and burning eyes!) For some people, *washable* mascara can hold on to a curl, but in most cases, it mascara goes on too wet and ends up undoing most of the curl.

Waterproof mascara also just lasts longer. If you want your mascara to look its best from morning until you wash your makeup off, try waterproof. Also, if you tend to cry or sweat easily, waterproof is for you.

The main complaint about waterproof makeup is that it can be difficult to remove when you're ready. There are some oil-free products that do a pretty good job removing waterproof makeup, but I still prefer an oil-based makeup remover, such as *Andrea Eye-Q's Makeup Remover Pads*. These work great but will leave an oily residue, so you have to follow them up with face wash.

* * *

RECOMMENDED MASCARAS

In my opinion (and no one is paying me to say this!) Maybelline makes the best mascaras. All of their mascaras come in washable and waterproof formulas.

Maybelline's Lash Sensational Mascara provides length and volume for a full fan effect. It's my favorite for people with medium to long lashes.

For people with shorter lashes, I recommend using a mascara that comes with a tiny brush so that you can access every little lash without making a huge mess all over your eye area. *Maybelline's Lash Discovery* is excellent for this reason. It's also great to use on bottom lashes.

* * *

HOW TO APPLY MASCARA

With mascara — like most endeavors in life — the more time you put into it, the better results you will get. But also like in life, if you are naturally blessed (like having thick, dark lashes) you might not need to do as much work. If your lashes are on the shorter, thinner side, and you want your eyes to stand out, be prepared to spend a few minutes here. No doing mascara at a red light for you!

After removing the mascara wand from the tube, scrape off any big globs onto the inside of the tube or on a tissue. Then, get the brush/wand as close to the base of your lashes as possible, and wiggle back and forth. Filling in the base of your lashes solidly with mascara creates the same effect as precisely-applied thin eye liner, therefore allowing us to skip eye liner altogether. (Yes, we will be skipping eyeliner in this book. We're all about maximum effectiveness here!)

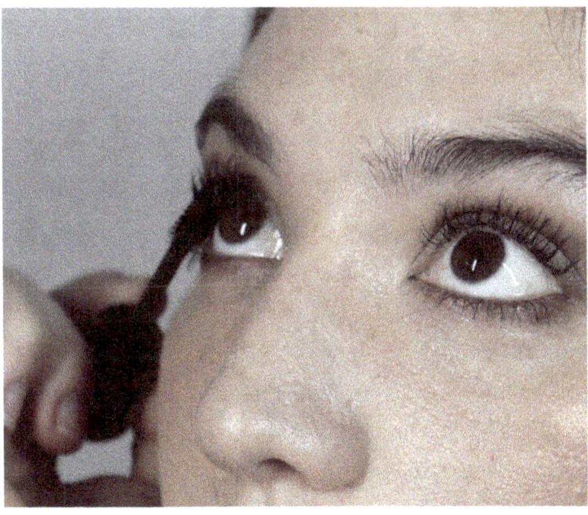

Once the base of your lashes is filled in, you can start coating the rest of the lashes. If you get some mascara on your skin, use a clean finger to wipe it off *right away* before it dries. After one coat, move on to your other eye, repeating the same process. After your second eye has its first coat, go back to the first eye for a second coat.

For the second coat, try to use the brush at different angles to reach the various sides of each lash. Turning the brush vertically can help you get to the side of each individual lash. If you have a strong curl, you can even swipe from above your lashes to coat the top side. Just remember to use a clean finger to quickly wipe off any smudges on your skin. Coating all sides of the lash does a much better job at creating the appearance of thick lashes than just swiping from underneath. And don't neglect the baby hairs in your inner and outer corners. Including those little ones has more effect than you would think!

CLEAN UP YOUR MESS

Now you will finally reap the benefits of starting with lashes first! After your vigorous mascara session, you may have made a mess on your eye lids, even if you tried wiping smudges off right away. Don't worry! Take a Q-Tip and swirl it in a bit of gentle eye cream such as *Cetaphil's Hydrating Eye Gel-Cream* or *CeraVe Skin Renewing Eye Cream* and rub it over any mascara smudges on your upper and lower lids until they are gone.

Important: Make sure you are using gentle lotion or eye cream for this clean-up step, *not makeup remover*. If you use makeup remover, the residue it leaves behind will dissolve the eyeshadow and concealer you'll be applying soon.

* * *

SHOULD YOU USE A LASH-ENHANCING SERUM?

If you wish your lashes were longer and maybe even thicker, and you're willing to be patient and spend a little money, lash serums are a great option. Lash serums are a thin liquid applied to your lash line, usually at night (although I have seen some brands that require you to do it morning and night). If you're diligent about adding it to your routine, you should start to see signs of longer lashes in about six weeks, with full effects after about three months. You have to continue using the product in order to maintain your results. Make sure to read about the side effects in advance. *GrandeLASH-MD* is a great option to try out first.

CHAPTER FIVE

Step 2: Eye Shadow

Aside from curling your lashes, using eyeshadow properly is one of the best ways to really accentuate your eyes! The goal of eye shadow is not necessarily to make your whole eye lid darker, but rather to use light and shade to create an illusion of sculpting your eyes into a more desirable shape, whether that means making them look bigger, more upturned, closer together, further apart, etc...

WHAT'S YOUR EYE SHAPE?

Most peoples' eyes fall into one of the following shape categories:

- Hooded
- Deep Set
- Monolid
- Prominent
- Almond

* * *

Knowing your eye shape can help you apply eyeshadow in a way that is most flattering for you. If you can't decide between two categories, it is not uncommon to fit into more than one category.

Also, after you determine your eye shape, you will next want to determine if your eyes fall into an additional sub-category.

* * *

HOODED

With hooded eyes, the fold of upper eyelid comes down very close to the upper lash line. In other words, the eyelid crease is very low. You can be born with hooded eyes, or your eyes can become hooded with age.

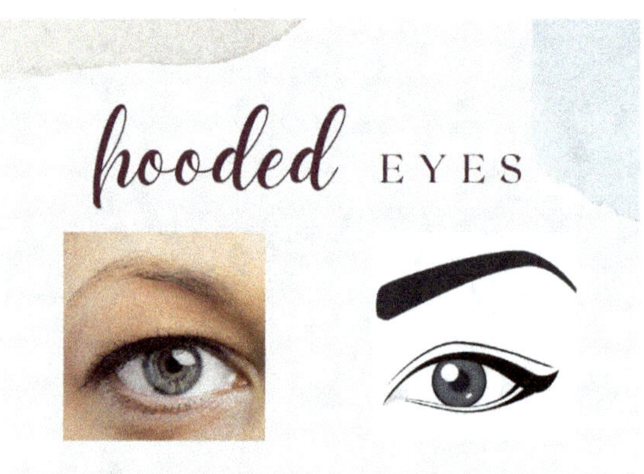

* * *

DEEP-SET

Deep-set eyes can sometimes be confused with hooded eyes, and sometimes people have both, especially as we age. With deep-set eyes, the brow bone comes out further than the eye.

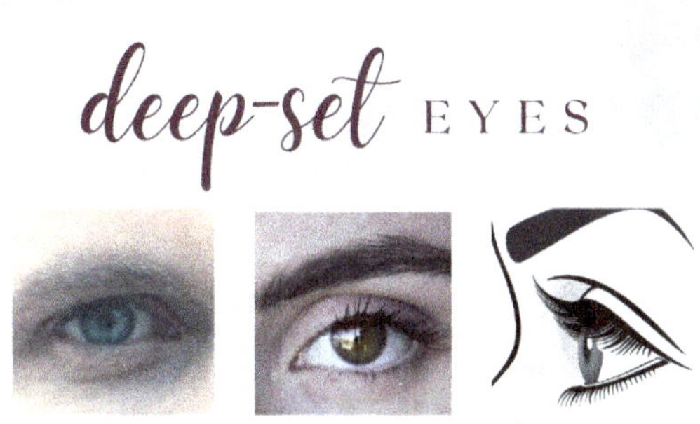

Deep-set eyes can sometimes be confused with hooded eyes, and sometimes people have both, especially as we age. With deep-set eyes, the brow bone comes out further than the eye.

PROMINENT (a.k.a. PROTRUDING)

Prominent eyes are the opposite of deep-set, coming out slightly further than the eye socket. Often prominent eyes have a crease in the lower eye lid.

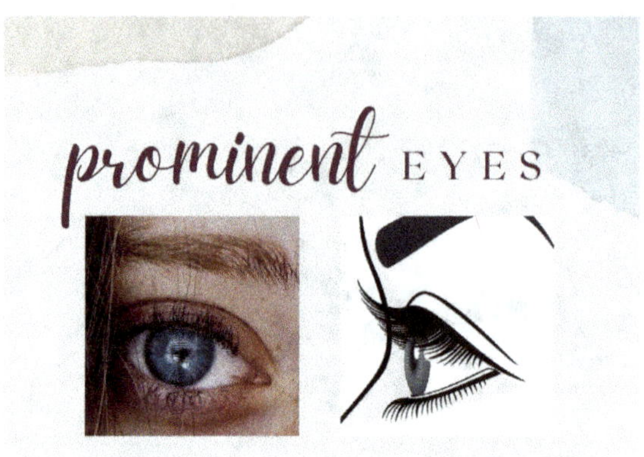

Prominent eyes are the opposite of deep-set, coming out slightly further than the eye socket. Often prominent eyes have a crease in the lower eye lid.

* * *

MONOLID

Monolid eyes are basically an extremely hooded eye. The crease comes all the way to the lash line, causing it to be barely visible, or not seen at all.

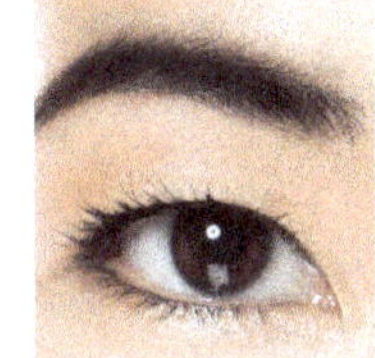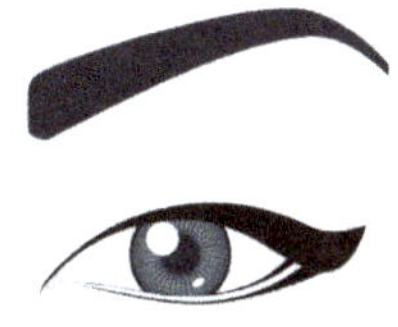

Monolid eyes are basically an extremely hooded eye.
The crease comes all the way to the lash line, causing
it not to be seen or barely visible.

* * *

ALMOND

If you don't feel like you fall into any of the other eye shape categories, you may have almond eyes. Almond-shaped eyes are essentially the average of all the other types.

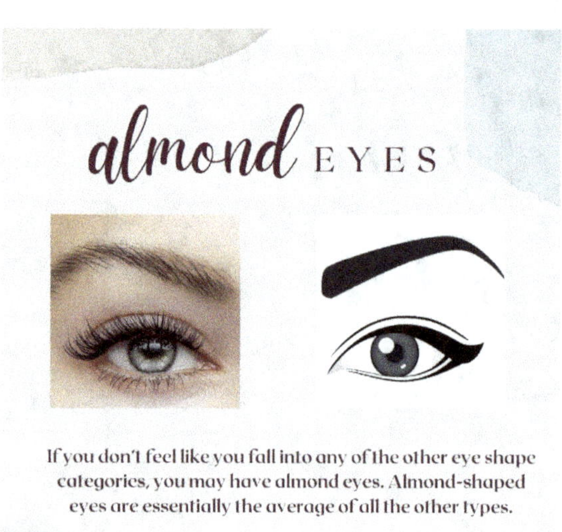

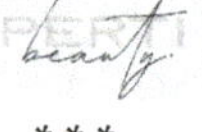

* * *

DO YOU HAVE AN EYE SUB-TYPE?

Sometimes, a person's eyes can fall into an additional category based on how the eyes are positioned. Standard eyes (i.e. normally-positioned eyes) are spaced about one eye-width apart, and the inner and outer corners are aligned. The following sub-types are for eyes that fall outside of that standard.

DOWN-TURNED EYES

For down-turned eyes, the top lash line curves down more than the bottom lash line curves up. The overall effect is that the eye is slanting downwards.

For down-turned eyes, the top lash line curves down more than the bottom lash line curves up. The overall effect is that the eye is slanting downwards.

* * *

WIDE-SET EYES

Wide-set eyes are more than one eye-width apart.

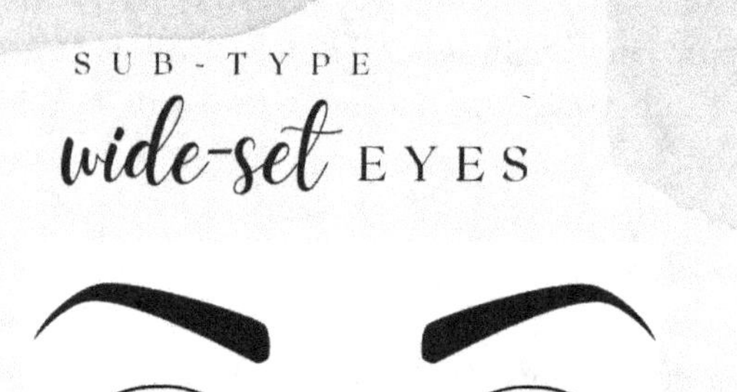

* * *

CLOSE-SET

Close-set eyes are less than one eye-width apart.

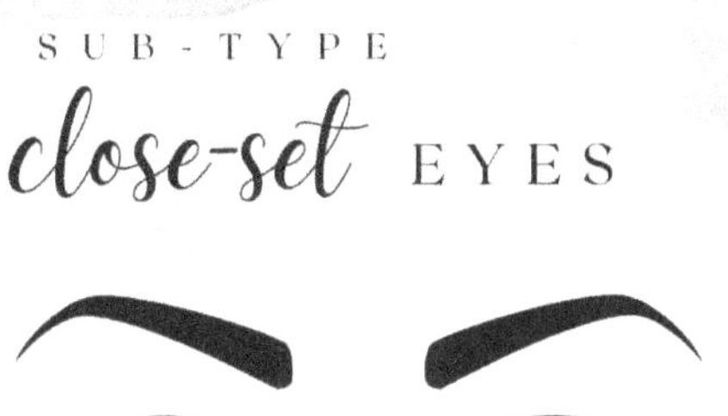

Close-set eyes are less than one eye-width apart.

* * *

A NOTE ABOUT EYE SHAPE

Almond-shaped and standard-set eyes are the *average* human eye shape, and therefore inherently balanced and appealing. We use makeup to create the illusion of balance, because evenness and symmetry are important components of aesthetic beauty. But please don't feel bad if you don't have almond-shaped, standard-set eyes! When people have features that fall out of the normal range, they are often considered *stunning*. In other words, one or more of their features stand out in such a way that other people stop in their tracks in admiration.

Many Hollywood stars and super-models have features that are anything but average. So if you have down-turned eyes, don't despair! So does Anne Hathaway. Hooded eyes? Zendaya, Blake Lively, and Jennifer Lawrence! And if you have prominent eyes, rejoice! So do Angelina Jolie and Mila Kunis! Monolid? Constance Wu and Lucy Liu! I could go on and on...

So despite the fact that balance plays a role in attractiveness, it is far from the only element involved in beauty. Don't be afraid to play up your uniqueness and stand out in your own way!

RECOMMENDED BRUSH SETS

Starting with this step, you will need your brushes. Buying brushes in a set is usually the most cost-effective option. *Morphe's Aurascape*, *Morphe's Travel Shape Essentials*, and *Real Techniques The Wanderer Makeup Brush Set* are all fantastic and affordable sets that each have everything you will need for the steps in this book. (You only need to purchase one of these sets.)

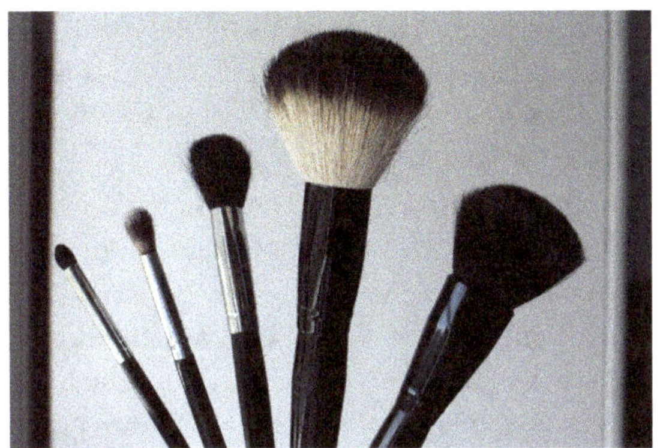

(Please note that these brushes are not from the kits
listed above, but they are the ones I used to complete the Six
Step Routine on my model.)

* * *

USING TWO COLORS OF EYESHADOW

With efficiency being a theme of this book, I'm going to show you how to accentuate your eyes using only two colors at a time. Just like illustrators use their pencils in different ways to create highlights and shadows, we will be using a lighter color and a darker color.

Try your best to choose colors that flatter your undertone. Refer back to the "Choosing Colors" chapter as needed.

For your lighter color, you will want to choose a color that is just a shade or two *lighter* than your skin tone. (Monolid eyes are the exception here. For your lighter color, choose one that is one shade *darker* than your skin tone.) If you want to incorporate shimmer in your eye look, do so with your lighter color. Use one of the small, flat shadow brushes from your set for this step.

For your darker color, choose a color that is 1-2 shades *darker* than your skin tone. (If you have monolid eyes, choose one that is 1-3 shades darker than what you chose for your lighter color.) The darker color should be matte (not have any shimmer.) Use a domed eye brush for this step. If you have a small eyelid area, use a smaller brush. You can choose a larger/fluffier brush if you have more eyelid space.

* * *

EYESHADOW RECOMMENDATIONS

Even, though this technique uses only two colors, I recommend buying an eye shadow palette so you can switch up your look as desired.

Here are my recommended eye shadow palettes. (These are the same as the ones I mentioned in the "Choosing Colors" chapter.)

Warm undertones — *NYX Professional Makeup Ultimate Color Shadow Palette in Warm Neutrals*

Cool undertones — *Morphe's 18CT Matte Essentials Artistry Palette*

Neutral undertones — *Colour Pop's 11:11 Pressed Powder Palette or Morphe's 18T Truth or Bare Artistry Palette*

HOW TO APPLY EYESHADOW FOR YOUR EYE SHAPE

APPLYING EYESHADOW TO HOODED EYES

APPLYING SHADOW TO
hooded EYES

1. Apply your lighter color from the lash line to the crease using a flat eyeshadow brush.
2. Apply the darker color from the crease up toward the eyebrow, but do not touch the eyebrow.
3. Use a fluffy eyeshadow brush to blend the transitions between the colors.

* * *

APPLYING EYESHADOW TO DEEP-SET EYES

* * *

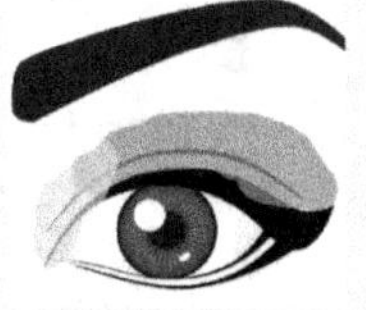
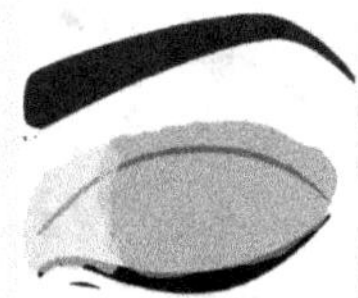
APPLYING SHADOW TO
prominent EYES
1. Apply your darker color on the outer two-thirds of your eyelid, from your lash line to a bit above the crease.
2. Apply your lighter color on the inner one-third of your eyelid.
3. Use a fluffy eyeshadow brush to blend the transition between the colors.

* * *

APPLYING EYESHADOW TO MONOLID EYES

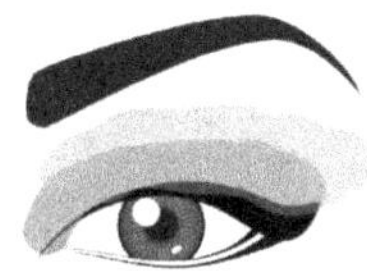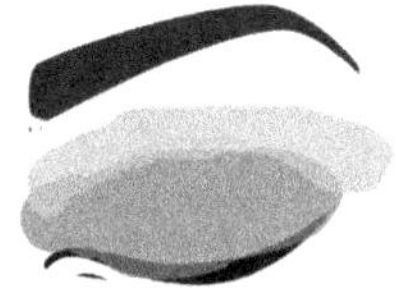

1. Apply your darker color along the lash line up to where you can feel your eyeball recede into the eye socket.
2. Apply your lighter color above this one.
3. Use a fluffy brush to blend the transitions between colors.

* * *

APPLYING EYESHADOW TO ALMOND EYES

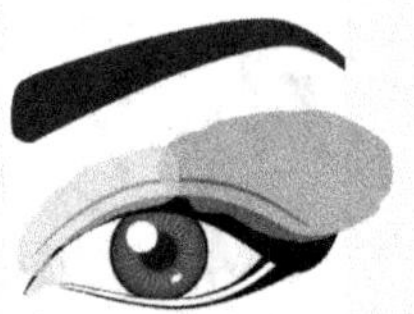
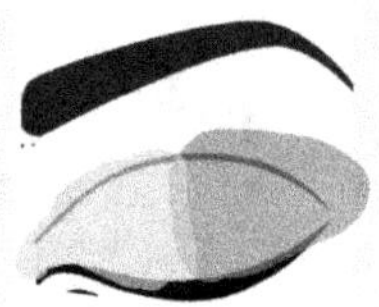

* * *

APPLYING EYESHADOW TO DOWN-TURNED EYES

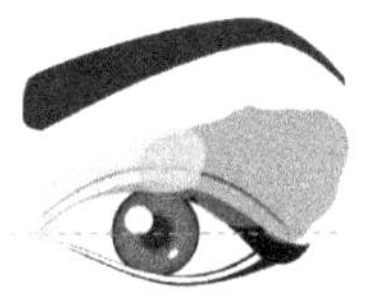
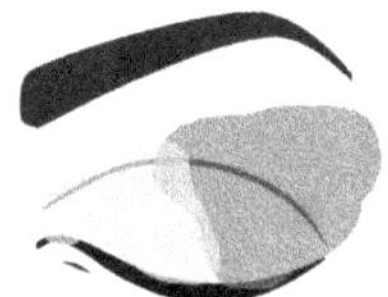

1. Apply the darker color on the outer half of the eyelid, curving up and out like a butterfly wing to visually lift.
2. Apply the lighter color on the inner half of the eyelid.
3. Use a fluffy eyeshadow brush to blend the transition area.

* * *

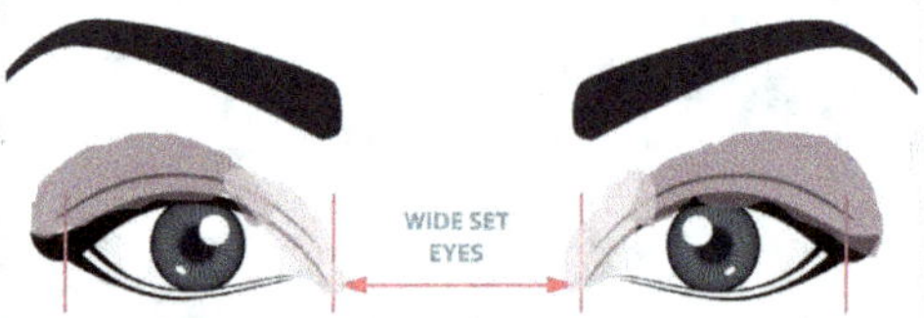

1. Apply the darker shade on most of the lid, from the lash line to above the crease. Do not go wider than the outer corner.
2. Apply the lighter color on the inner corners.
3. Blend with a fluffy eyeshadow brush in transition areas.

* * *

APPLYING EYESHADOW TO CLOSE-SET EYES

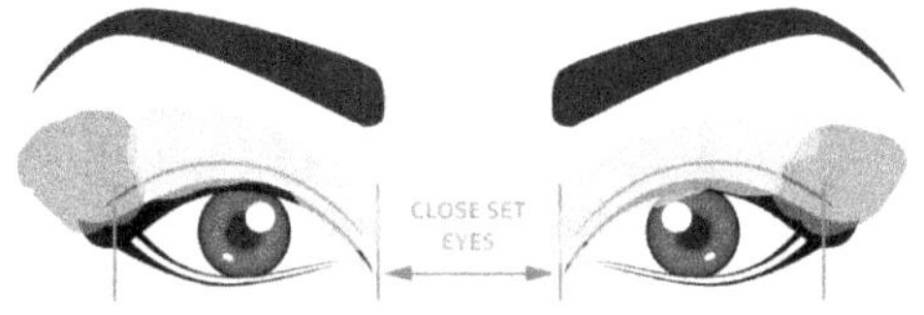

1. Apply the darker color on the outer one-third of the eyelid, from the lash line to above the crease.
2. Apply the lighter color on the inner two-thirds of the eyelid.
3. Use a fluffy eyeshadow brush to soften the transition between the colors.

* * *

EYESHADOW ON THE LOWER EYE-LID

If you want to thicken the appearance of your lower lashes and increase the appearance of your eyes overall, using eye shadow is a great option that doesn't look as jarring as bottom eyeliner! Using the small angled brush for your kit, use your darker shade to apply a line from your outer corner to about the middle of your eye. (Go closer to the inner corner for prominent or wide-set eyes.) Gently rub a finger tip at the stopping point to soften the transition.

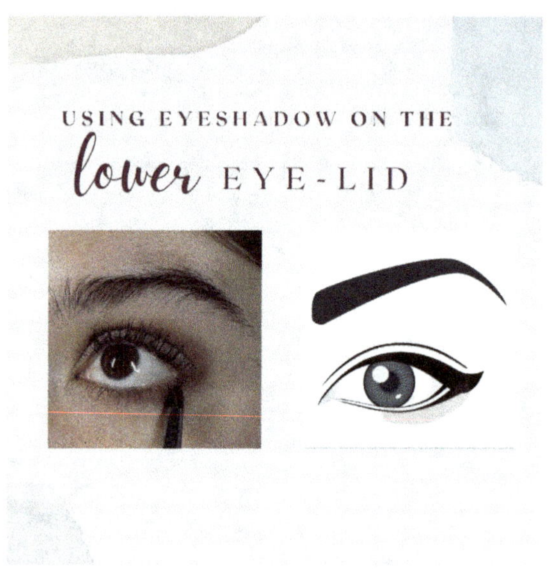

MAKE A MESS WITH YOUR EYESHADOW?

If you had a lot of dusting (a.k.a. *fallout*) from your eyeshadow onto your under-eye area or your cheeks, use a Q-Tip swirled in *Cetaphil* or *CeraVe* eye cream to clean it up like I recommended with the mascara. Since you have not applied foundation or concealer yet, you won't be ruining any of that work in the clean up process!

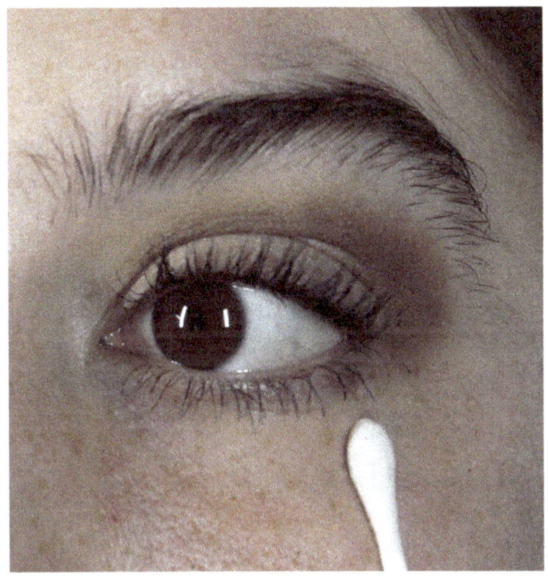

CHAPTER SIX

Step 3: Foundation

Foundation is a form of face makeup used to create an even base for the rest of your makeup. It serves as the groundwork for your entire makeup look, helping to even out skin tone, conceal imperfections, and provide a smooth canvas.

TYPES OF FOUNDATION

The number of foundations to choose from these days is seemingly endless, and many of them offer additional benefits. Of course, it's great to have options, but it can be overwhelming! Thankfully, most online makeup retailers have a way to filter your options by age, skin type, desired coverage level, finish, and other features you may want in your foundation. Here is an overview of each category.

FOUNDATION COVERAGE LEVELS

Coverage refers to how much of your own skin can be seen

through the foundation.

LIGHT-COVERAGE

A light-coverage foundation is nearly undetectable from your own skin. It will still show freckles, but won't completely cover discoloration or blemishes. Even though imperfections won't be completely covered, it still provides a subtle evening-out of skin tone.

MEDIUM-COVERAGE

Medium-coverage foundations cover minor imperfections, and even out skin tone nicely. When applied well, these foundations are not noticeable.

FULL-COVERAGE

Full-coverage foundations are thick and therefore easily conceal imperfections, but some formulas can look obvious if not applied with care.

* * *

FOUNDATION FORMULATIONS

The formulation of a foundation refers to it's ingredients and texture. Each of the three formulations have different properties that make them suitable for certain people over others.

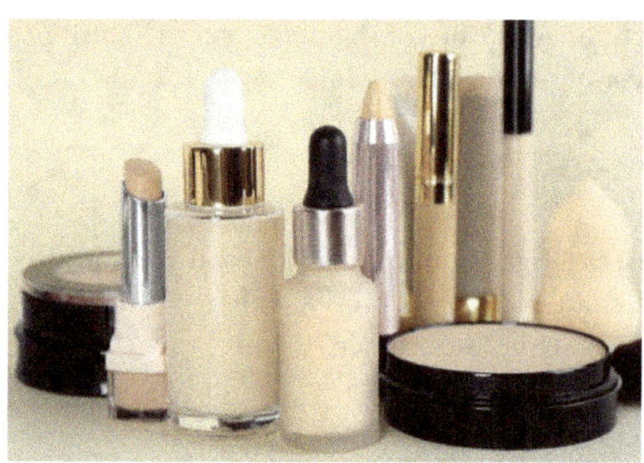

LIQUID FOUNDATIONS

The majority of foundations available are water-based liquid foundations. Liquid foundations offer build-able coverage, making them suitable for various occasions. They come in a variety of finishes, and can offer a variety of additional features. They can be applied with hands, brush, or sponge. BB Creams, tinted moisturizers, tinted primers, tinted SPFs, and serum foundations/tinted serums are all variations of liquid foundation given different names for marketing purposes.

CREAM FOUNDATIONS

* * *

Cream foundations are usually oil-based formulas mixed with skin-tone pigments. They leave a dewy finish with fuller coverage compared to powder and liquid foundations. They are less likely to dry out and settle into fine lines, so they are a great option for maturing skin. Due to their oil content, they may not be a great option for acne-prone skin.

POWDER FOUNDATIONS

Powder foundations are lightweight and often preferred by those who want a natural look. They work well for oily skin due to their matte finish. However, they can also be used in combination with liquid or cream foundations to add more coverage or to *set* the face.

FOUNDATION FINISHES

The finish of a foundation refers to how much light it absorbs or reflects.

DEWY

Dewy looks are often described as "luminous," "healthy," or "glowing." Dewy foundations use natural oils and humectants to reflect light, creating radiance and a youthful glow.

MATTE

A matte finish is characterized by an even, shine-free, and pore-less appearance, providing a velvety texture.

* * *

DEMI-MATTE

A demi-matte finish sits between dewy and matte. It's often referred to as "natural finish." If you want a foundation that provides natural-looking coverage with a hint of glow, this is a great option. Demi-matte foundations offer the long-wearing benefits of matte while maintaining a subtle luminosity, making them ideal for various skin types.

EXTRA FEATURES THAT FOUNDATION CAN HAVE

With so many competitors out there, makeup companies are constantly coming up with new ways to encourage people to buy their brand. For us, this means that foundations usually have several other benefits beyond smoothing out skin tone. Here are some examples of extras you can look for in your foundation:

- Long-wearing/transfer-resistant
- Waterproof
- Containing SPF
- Hydrating/moisturizing
- Anti-aging
- Acne-treating
- Hypoallergenic
- Vegan
- "Clean" — made without parabens, sulfates, phthalates, mineral oils, and other ingredients that have been shown to be harmful

* * *

FINDING YOUR FOUNDATION SHADE

After you've decided on a foundation, you will need to try find the shade that works best for you. The most effective way to do this is to buy your foundation from a store that allows you to test the products, such as Sephora, Ulta, and Blue Mercury. These stores usually have specially-trained employees who can help you decide.

In Sephora stores, you can ask an employee to do a Color IQ scan on your skin. This shade-matching technology will scan your skin for its color depth, undertone, and saturation, and then recommend products both in the store and on the website that would work for you.

If you can't make it to one of those stores, most drug stores will allow you to return beauty products even if they've been opened, as long as you have the receipt. Using this approach, you could buy a couple foundations that you think are close to your skin color and test them at home, in different kinds of lighting, especially outdoors. When testing foundation colors, swipe a line of each color along your jawline. This area is ideal because it typically has less color variation than the cheek area, and will help you choose a color that will transition nicely into your neck (which is almost always a different shade than our faces.) Whichever color is the most difficult to detect on your jawline will be your best match overall.

* * *

FOUR SEASONS OF FOUNDATION

Not only can our skin change color with the seasons, we may also want different finishes and coverage-levels as the seasons change. This section describes how to handle this 'season' issue in a cost-effective way.

If you have skin that changes color dramatically between seasons, adjusting your foundation as your skin changes is important. The simplest and most affordable way to do this is to have two foundation colors on hand. One color should be a match for your lightest winter skin, and the other for your tannest summer skin. In spring and fall, you can dispense a bit of each color onto your hand and mix them together to create a custom color that matches where you are on your own fair-to-tan spectrum.

You can also mix foundations together for other purposes, too, such as custom coverage-levels and finishes. Early in my makeup artist career, I made the mistake of ordering a slew of foundations for my kit without testing them! I had been pleased by that brand in the past so I assumed I would love that foundation. Unfortunately, I didn't love it. It was very high-coverage — way too much so for most of my clients — and it was very drying. Instead of ditching my $300 investment, I bought a few shades of a lightweight, dewy-finished foundation to mix with the drier foundations as needed. This allowed me to customize color, coverage, *and* finish for my clients in a way I would not have been able to before the mistake! Yay for happy accidents (and reading books for great advice!)

FOUNDATION RECOMMENDATIONS

* * *

Writing this section of the book has been daunting me the most, because there are so many incredible options out there these days. Keeping in mind that affordability is a theme of this book, however, here are my top suggestions for each skin type:

Combination/Normal: *about-face's THE PERFORMER Skin-Focused Foundation*

Dry: *ColourPop's Pretty Fresh Hyaluronic Hydrating Foundation*

Oily: *Revlon Colorstay 24 Hours Longwear Makeup*

Over 40: *Jones Road Beauty What the Foundation?* (This is more of a splurge, but I promise it's worth it. Foundation is the optimal place to spend a little more if you can.)

APPLYING FOUNDATION

There are so many options for applying foundations, but my overall favorite is… hands! In keeping with this book's theme of ease and cost-savings, I recommend applying foundation with your hands first. (This is assuming you chose a liquid foundation or a squeezable cream foundation. If you chose a stick or compact foundation, follow the instructions on the packaging, as it likely came with an applicator.)

I think hands are the best application tool, because:

- It is simple to ensure they are bacteria-free.
- They do not waste as much product as brushes and sponges.

- They create light to medium coverage.
- They can do the job fast with practice.
- They are easy to clean when you're done.

When you're ready to apply your foundation, make sure you start by washing your hands to remove any blemishing-causing bacteria. Then, dispense your foundation of choice into the palm of your non-dominant hand. If you need to mix in another foundation for custom-color/coverage/finish purposes, dispense the second one in your palm next to the first one, and use a finger to mix them together.

Using the product in your non-dominant palm, use your dominant hand to apply dots of foundation on your nose, forehead, cheeks, and chin. Then, using the foundation left on your fingers, start blending in the nose area and work your way outwards toward the hairline and jawline. Don't worry about getting it blended perfectly with your hands. Just make sure you get product wherever you want coverage.

Then, use a medium-to-large densely-bristled brush to buff it into your skin. Blend all over your face, but focus especially on transition areas such as your hairline, jawline, and eyebrows. Use the bit of product that the brush has picked up to transition your foundation color down into your neck for a seamless transition. We've all seen someone whose face and neck are totally different colors; this happens for two reasons. First, the foundation color they used was way off, and second, they did not blend well enough (or at all). You can get away with your foundation being off by a shade or even two as long as you are diligent about blending transition areas.

* * *

APPLYING *foundation*

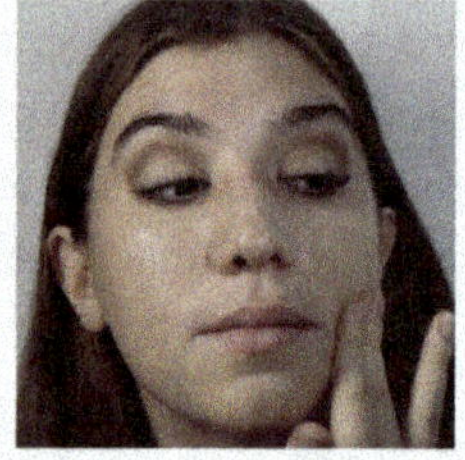

1. HANDS

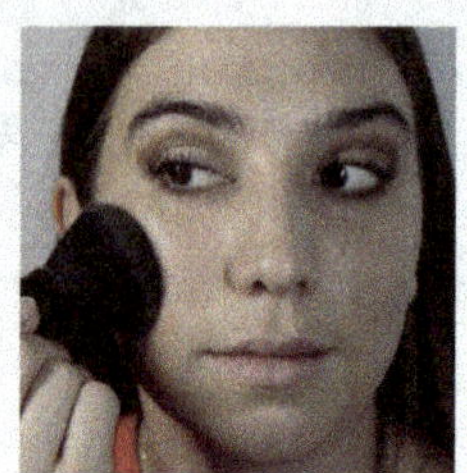

2. DENSELY-BRISTLED BRUSH

CHAPTER SEVEN

Step 4: Concealer

Concealer is specifically designed to cover localized imperfections on the skin. It targets areas with heavy-colored issues such as hyper-pigmentation, redness, dark circles, blemishes, acne and acne scars.

Sometimes people are surprised that I recommend applying concealer after foundation. There are two reasons. The first reason is that many lighter spots might be covered with foundation alone, so you would be wasting time applying concealer first. Secondly, if concealer is applied first, the process of blending the foundation into the skin might erase the work you did with the concealer.

CONCEALER TYPES AND RECOMMENDATIONS

Like foundations, concealers come in different formulas depending on what area you are trying to cover.

For dry and/or textured under-eye areas, a little bit of creamy concealer is a great option because it won't dry out and settle into fine lines. Two fabulous options are *IT Cosmetics Bye Bye Under Eyes or NUDESTIX NUDEFIX Cream Concealer*. (A little goes a long way with these products, so purchase the *mini* size to save yourself some money on these high-end brands!)

For concealing discolored areas on the face, you should opt for a formula that has the same finish as your foundation so the concealer doesn't catch light differently and look obvious. Additionally, you would not want to use a creamy, oil-based concealer on acne, which may exacerbate the acne. The cult-classic *Shape Tape Concealer* by *Tarte* works like a dream covering blemishes, and it can work beautifully covering dark eye circles on people with smooth and hydrated under-eye areas. It comes in a travel size that won't last you too long, but is great if you're trying it for the first time.

* * *

APPLYING UNDER-EYE CONCEALER

The pad of your ring finger is a great tool for applying and blending concealer under eyes, because it is just the right size and it's the weakest finger, so it is therefore the most gentle on this delicate area. Apply a dab of concealer to one ring finger and rub it against the other. Focus the product on the inner and outer corners, and tap your finger back and forth in gentle a stippling motion to blend. Remember to tap/dab/stipple! Do not rub or pull this delicate skin.

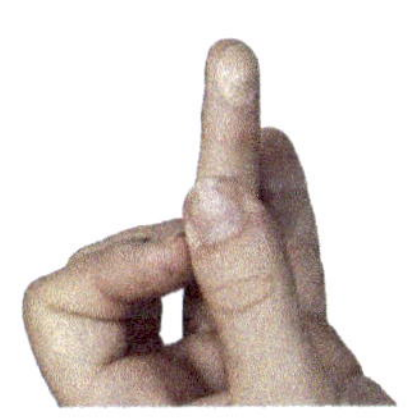

1. RING FINGER

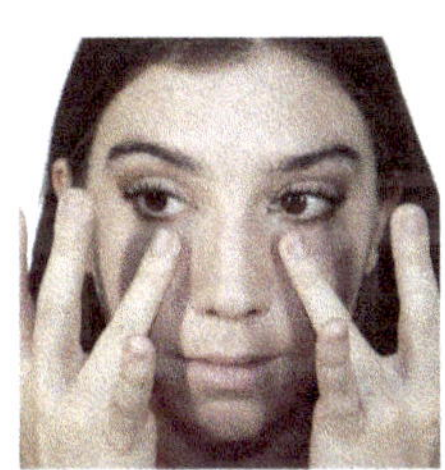

2. TAP BACK
AND FORTH
TO BLEND

SHOULD YOU USE A CORRECTOR TOO?

For the under-eye area, if you want a little extra help battling dark circles, you can use a corrector before the concealer. Under-eye correctors are usually a peachier color than concealers. The orangey-peach color of correctors helps to neutralize the purple-blue undertones of the under-eye area. *L.A. Girl Pro Conceal HD Concealer, Peach Corrector* is an effective, affordable option for light to medium skin tones.

Concealers on the other hand, come in the same range of colors as foundations, and should coordinate with your foundation so they blend together well. For double the under-eye coverage, start with a corrector and give it a few minutes to dry. Then apply a concealer on top.

APPLYING CONCEALER ON BLEMISHES

You can use finger tips to apply and blend concealer on other blemishes on the face as well. Still using a tapping/dabbing motion, focus the product directly on the spot you want to cover, and gradually move out from the spot in a spiral motion, so that there is a smooth transition from the spot into the rest of your foundation.

CHAPTER EIGHT

Step 5: Blush

In the name of evenness, foundation and concealer take the color out of our face and can make us look washed out. Fear not! That's where blush comes in! Bronzer is an option, too, which I will go over briefly in a later chapter.

TYPES OF BLUSH

Blush comes in powder and cream finishes, either matte or with shimmer.

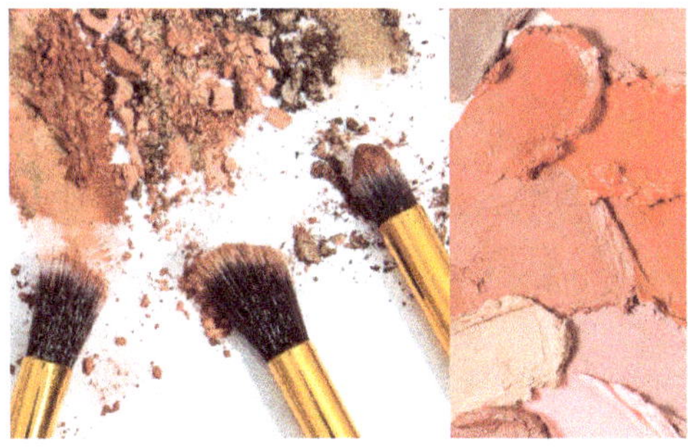

* * *

POWDER BLUSH

Powder blushes come in pressed powder form, and are suitable for normal, combination, or oily skin. They offer a longer-lasting effect than cream blushes. Powder blushes are best applied with a brush.

CREAM BLUSH

Cream blushes are emollient and come in tubes, wands, compacts, or twist-up sticks. They are great for dry skin as they provide hydration and a dewy finish. They can be a great choice for those with deeper skin tones due to their pigmentation and buildable color. Cream blushes are best applied with finger tips or sponges.

MATTE VS. SHIMMER BLUSHES

Both powder and cream formula blushes can come in matte or shimmer finishes. Which one you choose is mainly based on personal preference, although shimmer blushes can highlight uneven textures, so they're best to avoid if you have wrinkling, large pores, or acne scars in the cheek area.

BLUSH RECOMMENDATIONS

If you want to try a **cream blush** for its dewy, natural-flush effect, *Milani's Cheek Kiss Cream Blush* is a fabulous, budget-friendly option. *Milani* also has a three-color palette available for this formula.

If you're going for the classic, **powder blush**, here are the recommendations I made earlier, in the "Choosing Colors" chapter:

Warm undertones — *Milani's Baked Blush Luminoso* or *Rose D'Oro*

Cool undertones — *Milani's Baked Blush in Dolce Pink* or *Petal Primavera*

Neutral undertones — *Morphe's Complexion Pro Face Palettes* for fair (*8F*), medium (*8M*), tan (*8T*), rich (*8R*), and deep (*8D*) skin tones. Since people with neutral under

* * *

APPLYING BLUSH

I love cream blushes, but I do think proper use is a bit nuanced. It can be easy to overdo it with cream blushes. Also, and some what counter-intuitively, they don't have quite the lasting power that powder blushes have. So, for this book, I'm recommending powder blushes.

Imagine a line coming straight down from your pupil. Typically, we don't want to put any blush on the nose side of this line. Tap your blush brush into the product and apply it to the area just to the side of the imaginary line, opposite the nose. Tap, or *stipple*, your brush out towards your hairline.

As I write this book in 2024, the current blush trend is one that made me cringe at first, but has grown on me. The current trend is to start the blush a bit further from the nose and take it all the way up to the side of the eye. The thought is that this gives visual lift to the face. I have a feeling this is something we're going to laugh at in a few years, but for now, why not?

For a still-flattering and more classic look, keep your blush within the area outlined in the image below.

* * *

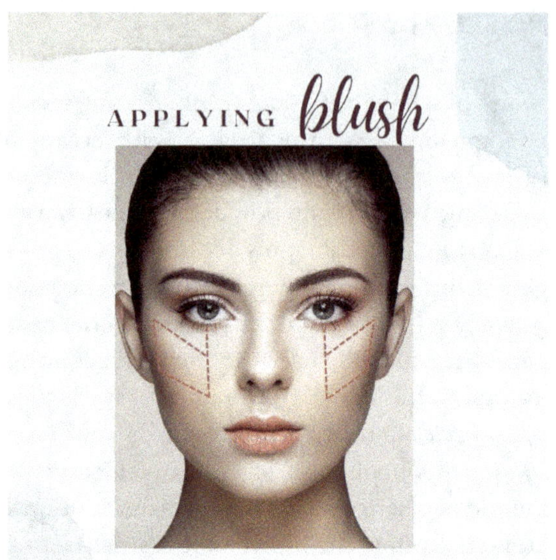

APPLYING blush

CHAPTER NINE

Step 5.5: Setting Powder (optional)

I'm referring to setting powder as Step 5.5 because it is optional, but it does have great benefits for some people.

BENEFITS OF SETTING POWDER

- Setting powder is great to use on top of foundation and concealer to lock them in place and help your makeup last longer.
- If you have oily or combination skin, setting powder can help control the shine.
- Setting powders can minimize the appearance of fine lines and large pores.
- Most setting powders will give a matte finish to your skin, so it can be used if you want to mattify a *dewy* or *demi-matte* foundation.
- Some setting powders include a very fine-milled shimmer, so these can be used to add a glowy effect to matte foundation, especially in the cheekbone area.

- Powder makeup can also be used over liquid or cream foundations to give added coverage.

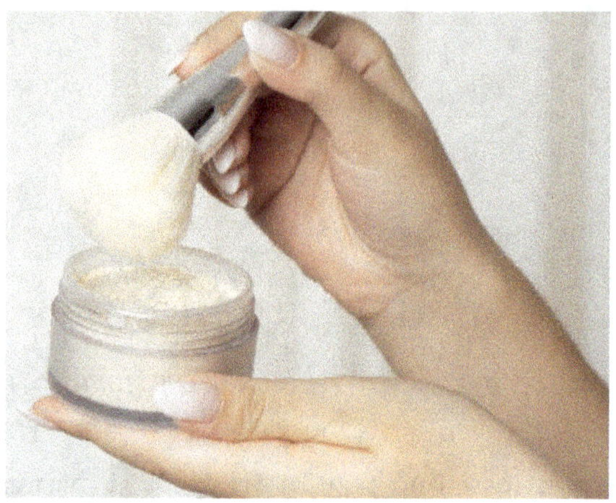

SETTING POWDER TYPES AND A RECOMMENDATION

Not all powders are labeled "setting powder" but pretty much any powder — *pressed* or *loose* — can be used to 'set' liquid or cream foundations, thereby extending the lasting-power of your makeup. In addition to being pressed or loose, powders can either have color or be translucent. Translucent powders look white in the package, but are see-through on the skin.

Morphe's Bake and Set Soft Focus Setting Powder is a great translucent, talc-free option.

* * *

APPLYING SETTING POWDER

Setting powders are often package with a sponge or puff applicator which can be used. Alternatively, loose setting powder can be quickly applied using a fluffy, loose-bristled makeup brush, and pressed powders can be applied with a more densely-bristled brush. Apply just enough to absorb shine. If you apply too much, you will look chalky.

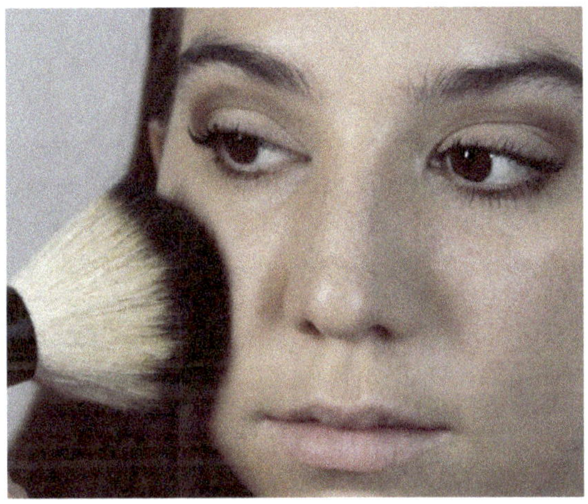

CHAPTER TEN

Step 6: Lip Color

I'll be honest, I am personally not much of a lip color user in my day-to-day mom/writer life. Most times, if I have anything on my lips, it is probably *Aquaphor Lip Repair* — the squeezy tube one (I don't find the roll-up tube to be as moisturizing). And even when I do wear a lip color, I prefer neutrals that are close to my natural lip color. But — some people love lip color and wear it all the time — even when alone — because it just makes them feel better! It is really a personal choice that often depends on your plans for the day. Adding color to your lips is great for looking your best for first-impression and arrival scenarios. It simply pulls your whole look together like a cherry on a sundae!

CHOOSING A COLOR FOR YOUR LIPS

When choosing a color for your lips, make sure to color-coordinate your lip color with the rest of your makeup, as discussed in the "Choosing Colors" chapter. It's hard to go

wrong with a color that is just a shade or two deeper than
your natural lip color.

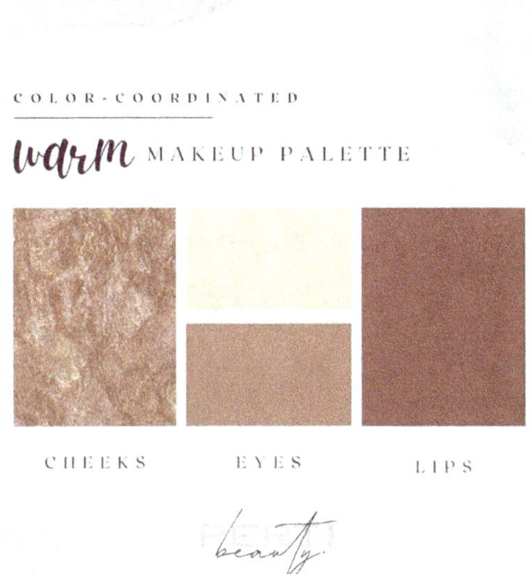

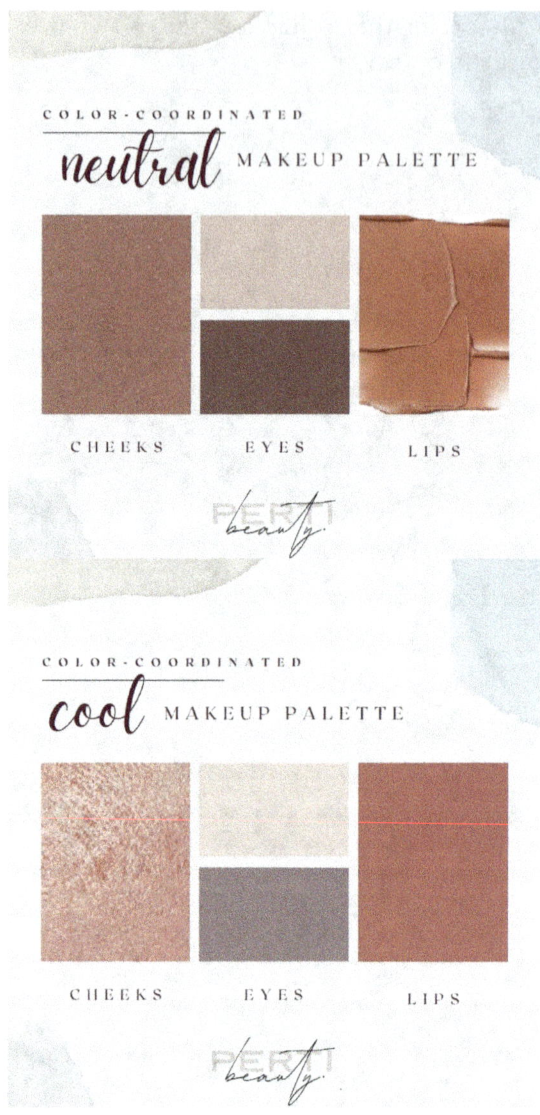

If you plan on wearing a bold lip color, it is generally

recommended to go lighter on your eye and cheek colors to avoid looking overdone, especially during the day. (This 'rule' can be broken for a nighttime party look, especially if you know you will be in dim lighting. And any 'rule' can be broken for self-expression purposes!)

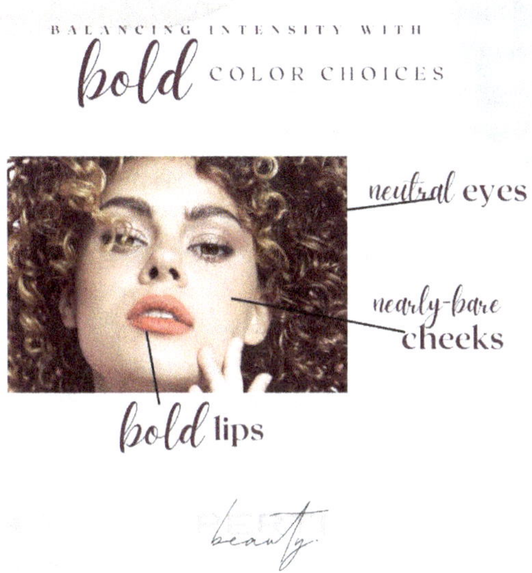

MAKEUP FOR PHOTOS

If you want to look your best in photos, lip color is a great idea. Makeup artist dogma states that photos "take off" 50% of makeup. In other words, makeup looks less intense in photographs than it does in real life. I don't know how legit that 50% statistic is, but it's a good rule of thumb to keep in mind. So, if you are doing makeup exclusively for a photography session, you can apply everything more heavily than you would if your main goal is to look good in person.

If you're doing makeup for an in-person event where there will be many pictures taken, such as prom or a wedding, my advice is this: apply makeup that you are happy with in the mirror, then bit by bit, go bolder with your eye, cheek, and lip color, testing your look in photos as you go. This will help you find the delicate balance that looks beautiful in person and in pictures.

LIP COLOR TYPES AND RECOMMENDATIONS

Just like foundations and cheek colors, lip colors come in a variety of formulations and finishes that are ideal for different purposes.

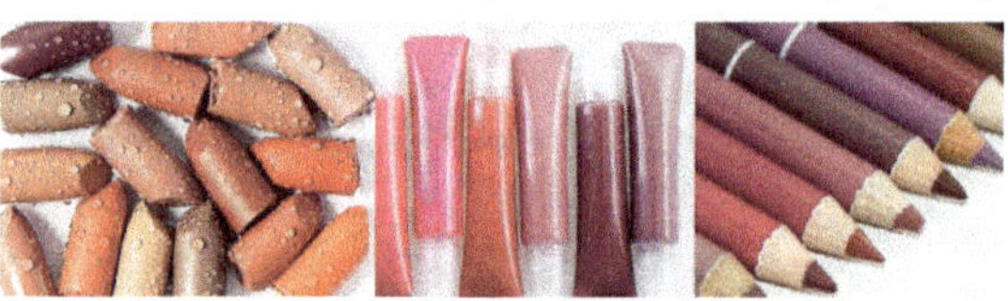

LIP GLOSS

Lip gloss adds shine and the appearance of fullness to lips. They can be clear or have color. Color lip glosses are translucent which means they give great shine and can also have bit of color. Because they are translucent, lip glosses don't need to be applied with precision — they just follow the natural contours of your lips. For this reason, they are easy to use for touch ups because you don't even need a mirror! The downside of lip glosses is that they don't last long. There are more viscous (i.e. sticky) glosses that can last about two hours, but many people don't care for the stickiness.

Maybelline's Lifter Gloss comes in several beautiful colors is formulated with hyaluronic acid to give lips a fuller look and a hydration boost.

LIPSTICK

You know what lipstick is, right? Probably, but I'm going to tell you anyway. Traditional lipstick is a solid made of wax and oil that comes in a twist-up tube in an endless array of colors. Lipsticks can be matte, creamy, or glossy.

Here is something you might *not* know about lipstick! Lipstick dates back to ancient peoples such as the Sumer, Indus Valley, and Egyptian civilizations. Both men and women used crushed gemstones, bugs (such as carmine), and other natural materials to decorate their lips. In ancient Egypt, lip coloring was associated with social status rather than gender.

If you don't feel like putting crushed bugs on your lips, *E.L.F. O FACE Satin Lipstick* is a highly-rated and affordable option.

LIQUID LIPSTICK

Liquid lipstick has the rich, opaque look of traditional lipstick with the tube-and-wand application method of a lip gloss. They come in a variety of finishes. I am a big fan of *Milani's Amore Shine and Amore Satin Matte Lip Color* lines. They come in a range of gorgeous, flattering colors and are budget-friendly!

LIP STAIN

* * *

Lip stain is color that seeps into the skin of the lips for long-lasting, transfer-resistant color with a natural finish. Lip stains are usually not as opaque as lipsticks or liquid lipsticks. They can be layered with gloss to give the appearance of fuller lips.

I've recently tried *WONDERSKIN's Wonder Blading Lip Stain Masque,* and I'm obsessed! It goes on blue but when you wipe the blue off, your lips are left with a gorgeous, naturally-textured flush. The color selection is great, too!

ColourPop Ultra Blotted Lip is a popular option that's cross between liquid lipstick and a stain.

PREPARING YOUR LIPS FOR COLOR

It's a great idea to gently exfoliate your lips before applying color to help the product go on smoothly. You can do this easily with a toothbrush! After brushing your teeth, rinse your toothbrush and gently brush your lips! Doing this regularly once a day will keep your lips nice and smooth.

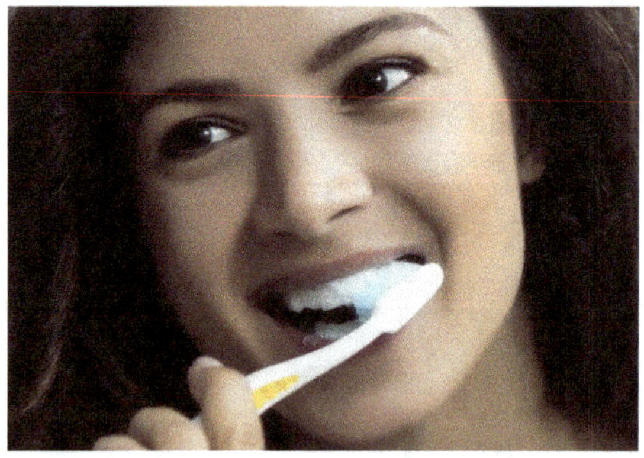

LIP LINER

* * *

Lip liner is optional, but it's helpful for adding the appearance of fullness to lips and for creating crisp outlines when using a bold color.

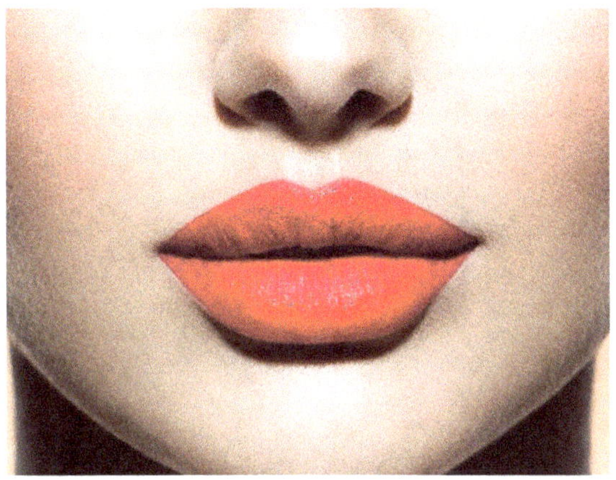

HOW TO APPLY LIP COLOR

APPLYING LIP LINER

If you're using lip liner solely to create crisp edges for a bold lip color, you can draw an outline around your lips. Be careful to make sure the sides are symmetrical. It will take practice to get it perfect, but it's worth it if you like bold colors. When you're done outlining, smudge the color a bit so that you're not left with a clownish outline if your lipstick fades faster than your lip liner.

If you're using lip liner to add fullness to your lips, there is an ideal way to do this. First, instead of following your natural lip line, you will want to *over-line* your lips. Use the lip liner just slightly outside of the lines of your natural lips, by about as much as the width of the liner tip. Second, do not line all the way into the corners. Instead, taper the line in towards your mouth before you reach the corners, on the top and bottom.

Try *NYX Professional Makeup Line Loud Longwear Lip Liner* for smooth, transfer-proof color.

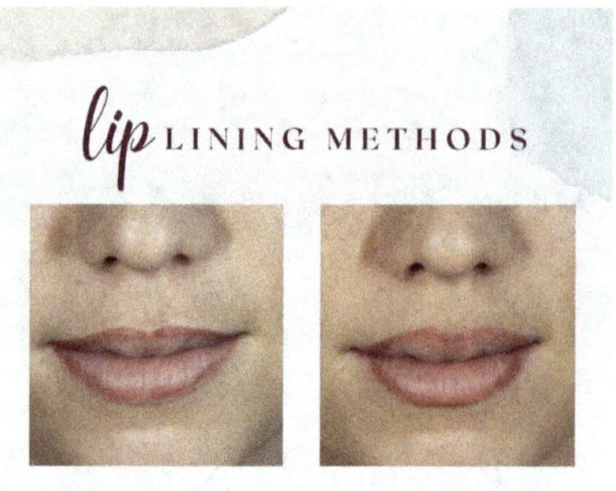

Basic Outlining vs. Lining for Fullness

* * *

APPLYING LIP COLOR

How you apply lip color depends on which type you are using, but is pretty self-explanatory. The main thing I want to note about lip color, is that applying layers will help with lasting power. To help lip color last as long as possible:

1. Use lip liner.
2. Use a long-lasting formula lip color to fill in the rest of the area.
3. Blot, then press translucent setting powder into the lip color with a finger tip.
4. Apply a second coat on top of the first coat.

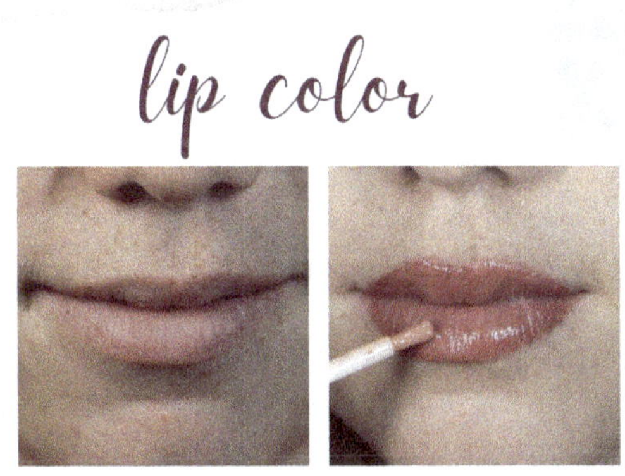

BEFORE   VS.   AFTER

CHAPTER ELEVEN

Optional Finishing Touches

Here are a few more things you may find helpful regularly or on occasion.

MAKE IT LAST

To help your whole makeup look last longer, finish with a setting spray to lock in your makeup. Setting sprays come in a variety of finishes such as mattifying/oil-controlling, natural-finish, and dewy. A great and affordable oil-controlling option is *L.A. Girl PRO Perfect Oil Control Multitasking Setting Spray*.

Close your eyes, hold the spray about eight inches away from your face, and spray away. This may make you face feel wet, which might freak you out at first. But it will dry in a couple minutes, and your hard work will have an extra layer of invisible protection.

* * *

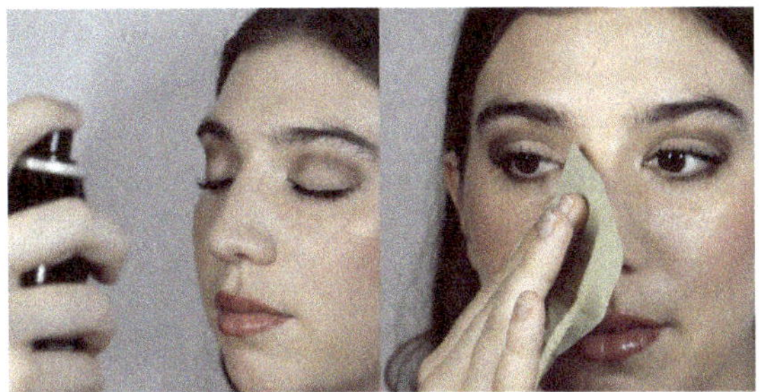

TOUCH UPS

If you follow the recommendations in this book and aren't participating in a triathlon, the only touch-ups you might need will be re-applying lip color and absorbing any break-through shine.

If you experience shine, that doesn't necessarily mean your makeup is gone. You can absorb the shine without messing up your makeup or applying more by pressing blotting papers to the oily areas, such as *NYX PROFESSIONAL MAKEUP Matte Blotting Papers*.

EYEBROWS

Eyebrow styling and makeup could almost be a whole book, because eyebrow trends change every few years. In this book, I have focused on covering timeless makeup tips. So, I'm not including brows other than to say that clear brow gel (like *NYX PROFESSIONAL MAKEUP The Brow Glue*) is a quick, versatile, fool-proof option for many people. Brow gel can be used to either tame your brows into a more streamlined look, or to style them in a way that makes them look fuller.

Brow serum is a great option for adding new growth to sparse eyebrows.

Brow tinting is helpful if you do have brow hairs, but they are too light.

Permanent makeup techniques such as *microblading, microshading, ombré brows,* etc… are an option if your brows are chronically spare and you like a defined brow look. Just make sure to do lots of research before to committing to this process, because it is essentially a tattoo and may never fade completely.

CHAPTER TWELVE

The 6-Steps Cheat Sheet

Refer to this graphic to help you remember the steps until your new routine becomes second nature! Make sure to read the preceding chapters for help with choosing the right products and colors, and important how-to information.

* * *

Pretty in a Pinch
6-Step Makeup Routine

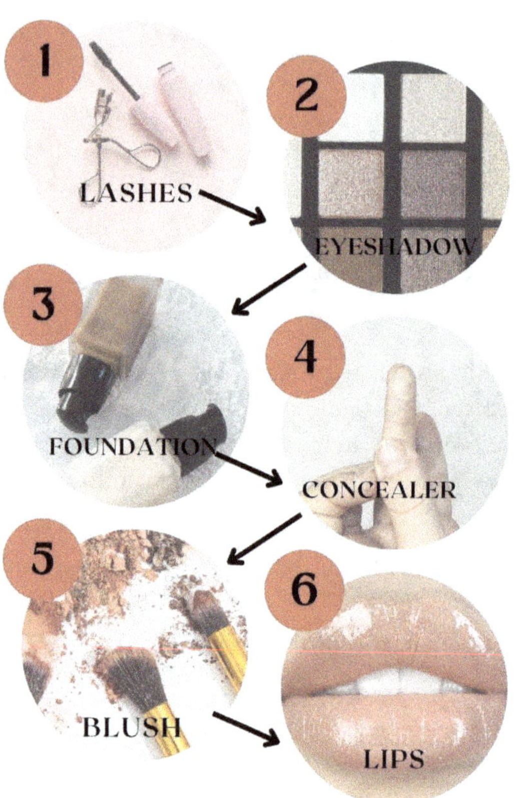

CHAPTER THIRTEEN

What's Not in the 6-Steps

What about primers, eye liner, bronzer and contouring?

These things all have their place, but I didn't include them because I don't think they are necessary for a quick, everyday, pretty look. But in case you were really hoping to learn a bit about these, here's a very brief overview.

PRIMERS

Primers prepare your skin to help makeup go on smoothly and last longer. If you take care of your skin and apply a moisturizer before your foundation, your skin is primed! You can buy specialty primers to use on top of your moisturizer if you're especially concerned about oil-control or increasing your makeup's lasting-power.

BRONZERS

* * *

Bronzers are a warm-toned product applied on top of foundation to help achieve a sun-kissed look. They can be used instead of or in addition to blush. Powder bronzers are most common and most convenient to use. They should be applied lightly to the areas of the face that would typically get color if you'd been out in the sun, such as forehead, nose, and upper cheek area.

CONTOURING

Contour products are cool-toned powders or creams that are used to help create subtle shadows in strategic areas of the face, thereby shaping the face. They can be used to accentuate cheekbones, visually slim the face, nose, and jawline, as well as create the illusion of a smaller forehead or chin.

If you want to play around with contouring, I find powder contouring to be easier and more forgiving than cream contouring. However, cream contouring is more dramatic and effective at creating the appearance of a sculpted face, especially in photographs. Cream contour can look a little heavy for in-person looks. You can look online for facial contouring maps and directions, but it is more of an advanced skill, which is why I left it out of this book.

CHAPTER FOURTEEN

Have fun!

If you're completely new to makeup, I can imagine that this all feels overwhelming. Maybe it's even overwhelming if you are familiar with makeup. That's OK. I tried to find a balance between what would be useful, novel information but not superfluous. To make getting started simpler, consider focusing on learning one step at a time.

Or, if you're more excited than overwhelmed, just bite the bullet and clear an hour or so from your schedule to try all the steps at once! With practice, all six steps should only take about ten minutes, believe it or not, because so much of the content of this book was about choosing the right products and colors for your needs. Once the task of choosing everything is out of the way, it's all about the application process and having fun!

If you find the tips in this book helpful, please consider taking a minute to help me out by leaving a happy-customer review on Amazon.

With that, I'll leave you with this quote by renowned

makeup artist, Kevyn Aucoin:

> "I'm not saying that putting on makeup will change
> the world or even your life, but it can be a first step
> in learning things about yourself you may never
> have discovered otherwise. At worst, you could
> make a big mess and have a good laugh."

(And if you do make a big mess… you've got Q-Tips dipped
in eye cream to clean it up!)

CHAPTER FIFTEEN

References

The following sources assisted with the content creation of this book:

Hopp, D., & Rostamian, M. (2024, January 4). How to identify your skin undertone, according to makeup artists. *Byrdie.* https://www.byrdie.com/figure-out-undertones

How to identify your undertones. (n.d.). Revlon. https://www.revlon.com/editorial-content/how-to-identify-your-undertones

Skincare, O. C. C. C. C. +. O. (n.d.). *Cool, warm or neutral: understanding skin tones + undertones.* Orglamix Clean Consciously Crafted Cosmetics + Organic Skincare. https://orglamix.com/pages/cool-neutral-or-warm-best-shade-mineral-foundation-natural-mineral-makeup

Maestra, B. (2023, February 28). *What is foundation makeup? The 5 main types and benefits.* The Beauty Maestra. https://thebeautymaestra.com/makeup/what-is-foundation-makeup/

Paris, L. (2024, February 15). *what-is-foundation-makeup*. L'Oréal Paris. https://www.lorealparisusa.com/beauty-magazine/makeup/face-makeup/what-is-foundation-makeup

Wikipedia contributors. (2024, April 26). *Foundation (cosmetics)*. Wikipedia. https://en.wikipedia.org/wiki/Foundation_%28cosmetics%29

Zahid, N. (2024, February 17). *Foundations 101: The Ultimate guide to flawless makeup*. Belle Beauties. https://www.bellebeauties.com/foundations/

Noble, A. (2022, December 22). Cream vs. Liquid vs. Powder Foundation: When to Use Each One. *InStyle*. https://www.instyle.com/cream-vs-liquid-vs-powder-foundation-6890626

Manager, T. B. a. C. (2022, March 9). *How to choose the right powder, liquid or cream foundation*. NewBeauty. https://www.newbeauty.com/need-to-know-about-powder-vs-liquid-makeup/

Tucker, A. (2017, June 22). *Should you use liquid, cream, or powder makeup? Here's what you need to know*. Bustle. https://www.bustle.com/p/should-you-use-liquid-cream-powder-makeup-heres-what-you-need-to-know-63919

Hickman, J. M. (2018, December 17). StyleCaster. *StyleCaster*. https://stylecaster.com/beauty/makeup/467146/how-to-find-right-foundation-finish/

Sowerbutts, K. (2023, July 20). *A Foolproof guide to foundation finishes - Beauty Bay edited*. Beauty Bay Edited. https://www.beautybay.com/edited/foundation-finishes/

Savini, L. (2023, February 15). *Cream Blush vs. Powder Blush: We Asked Makeup Artists to Settle the Debate*. Byrdie. https://www.byrdie.com/cream-vs-powder-blush-7109582

Team, C. (2023, July 6). Cream vs. powder: The definitive guide to blush. *Curology*. https://curology.com/blog/cream-vs-powder-the-definitive-guide-to-blush/

Jackson, K. (2023, May 3). *Cream Blush Vs. Powder Blush — Which is Best for You?* The Makeup Refinery. https:// themakeuprefinery.com/cream-or-powder-blush/

How is cream blush different from powder blush? - into the gloss. (2016, February 12). Into the Gloss. https://intothegloss.com/ beauty-advice/how-is-cream-blush-different-from-powder-blush/

Wikipedia contributors. (2024b, May 27). *Lipstick.* Wikipedia. https://en.wikipedia.org/wiki/Lipstick

Ross, S. (2024, April 3). *55 makeup quotes any Beauty-Lover can relate to.* Byrdie. https://www.byrdie.com/makeup-quotes-4768957